EVERYTHING ABOUT LUNG CANCER DIET

A Comprehensive Guide To Nutritional Strategies, Foods To Avoid, Healing Recipes For Optimal Health And Recovery

WALTON USELTON

© 2024 [WALTON USELTON]

All rights reserved. No part of this book may be reproduced, distributed, or transmitted in any form or by any means, including photocopying, recording, or other electronic or mechanical methods, without the publisher's prior written permission, with the exception of brief quotations in critical reviews and certain other noncommercial uses permitted by copyright law.

DISCLAIMER

The content in this book is based on the author's expertise and understanding of food and nutrition. The author is not linked or associated with any corporation, business, or person. This book is designed for informative purposes only and should not be interpreted as professional medical advice. Readers should get medical advice before making any changes to their diet or lifestyle. The author takes no responsibility or liability for any repercussions arising from the use of the information included in this book.

Table of Contents

INTRODUCTION 9

An Overview OF Lung Cancer AND Its Effect ON Health 9

Importance Of Diet In Managing Lung Cancer .. 10

Lung Cancer Diet Goals 11

   1. Support General Health: 11

   2. Manage Symptoms and Side Effects: 11

   3. Optimise Treatment results: 11

   4. Reduce the Risk of problems: 12

Basic Nutritional Principles For Cancer Patients 12

   1. Eat a Variety of Nutrient-Rich Foods: 12

   2. Remind Hydrated: 12

   3. Maintain a Healthy Weight: 13

   4. Manage Side Effects: 13

   5. Consult a Registered Dietitian: 13

How to Use This Book Effectively 14

   1. Study Each Section Carefully: 14

   2. Apply the advice: 14

CHAPTER ONE 17

Understanding Lung Cancer 17

Types And Stages Of Lung Cancer 17
    Types of Lung Cancer 17
    Stages of Lung Cancer 18
Common Symptoms And Diagnostic Methods .. 19
    Symptoms Of Lung Cancer 19
    Diagnosis Methods: 20
Treatment Alternatives And Side Effects 21
    Treatment Options: 21
    Side Effects 22
The Role Of Nutrition In Cancer Care 23
    Importance of Nutrition 23
    Nutritional recommendations 23
Myths And Facts On Lung Cancer And Diet 25
    Myth: Sugar Fuels Cancer Cells. 25
    Fact: Balanced nutrition is key. 25
    Myth: Alternative treatments can cure cancer.
    .. 26
    Fact: Complementary Approaches Can Help
    Treat 26
CHAPTER TWO 27
    Nutritional Needs Of Lung Cancer Patients 27

Macronutrients Include Proteins, Carbohydrates, And Fats 27

Micronutrients Include Vitamins And Minerals 28

Importance Of Hydration 30

Caloric Needs And Energy Balance 31

Adjusting Nutritional Needs During Treatment 32

CHAPTER THREE 35

High-Protein Foods For Muscle Maintenance 35

Fruits And Vegetables With High Antioxidant Levels 36

Whole Grains And Their Benefits 37

Healthy Fats: Their Sources 37

Hydrating Foods And Beverages 38

CHAPTER FOUR 41

Foods To Avoid 41

Processed And Red Meats 41

Sugary Beverages And Snacks 42

Excessive Salt And Sodium-Rich Foods 43

Alcohol And Its Effects On Therapy 44

Artificial Additives And Preservatives 44

CHAPTER FIVE 47
Menu Planning And Preparation 47
Creating Balanced Meal Plans 47
Quick & Easy Recipes 48
Tips For Meal Prep And Storage 50
1. Plan Ahead: 50
3. Use Freezer-Friendly Containers: 50
4. Preparing Ingredients in Advance: 51
5. Consider Convenience Foods: 51
Adjusting Meals For Side Effects 51
Incorporating Family And Cultural Preferences 52

CHAPTER SIX 55
Supplements And Alternative Therapies 55
Role Of Dietary Supplements 55
Popular Supplements For Cancer Patients 57
Assessing The Safety And Efficacy Of Supplements 59
Alternative Diets And Therapies 61
1. Ketogenic Diet: 61
2. Vegan Diet: 61

4. Mind-Body Therapies: 62
Consulting With Healthcare Providers 63
CHAPTER SEVEN 65
Managing Side Effects Via Diet 65
Addressing Nausea And Vomiting 65
Coping With Taste And Smell Changes 66
Strategies To Manage Appetite Loss 67
Dealing With Diarrhoea And Constipation 68
Foods That May Help With Mouth Sores And Difficulty Swallowing 70
CHAPTER EIGHT 73
Emotional And Psychological Support 73
Effects Of Diet On Mental Health 73
Strategies To Stay Motivated 74
Creating A Support Network 75
Stress Management Techniques 76
Mindful Eating And Its Benefits 77
CHAPTER NINE 79
Exercise And Physical Activity 79
Benefits Of Exercise For Lung Cancer Patients .79
Types Of Suitable Physical Activities 80

Incorporating Exercise Into The Daily Routine 81
Balancing Activity, Rest, And Recovery 82
Working With Physical Therapists And Trainers
.... 83
CHAPTER TEN 85
Long-Term Dietary Strategies 85
Maintaining A Healthy Weight 85
Preventing Cancer Recurrence With Diet 86
Establishing A Lifelong Healthy Eating Pattern 87
Regular Follow-Ups With A Dietitian 88
Diet Changes To Meet Changing Health Needs..89
CONCLUSION 91
THE END 93

ABOUT THIS BOOK

"Lung Cancer Diet" is an important handbook that emphasizes the importance of diet in the prevention and treatment of lung cancer. It starts with an interesting introduction that explains how lung cancer affects general health and emphasizes the importance of food in controlling this illness. This book establishes clear objectives for a lung cancer diet and outlines the fundamental nutritional concepts that are specially targeted to cancer patients. This introduction part also includes helpful tips on how to browse and use This book efficiently.

Understanding lung cancer is critical, and This book digs fully into its many forms and stages, typical symptoms, and diagnostic tools. It investigates numerous treatment choices and their related side effects, focusing on how diet might help alleviate these adverse effects and improve patient results. The work dispels prevalent beliefs and gives facts concerning the link between lung cancer and food, resulting in a better knowledge of the condition.

A large amount of this book is devoted to the dietary requirements of lung cancer patients. It includes detailed information on macronutrients like proteins, carbs, and fats, as well as micronutrients such as important vitamins and minerals. The need for water is emphasized, as is thorough information on calorie requirements and energy balance, particularly throughout treatment stages when nutritional demands may alter.

This book then shifts to practical dietary recommendations, outlining the sorts of foods that are good for lung cancer sufferers. High-protein diets are advised for muscle maintenance, as well as antioxidant-rich fruits and vegetables to prevent oxidative stress. The advantages of whole grains, healthy fats, and hydrating meals and drinks are also carefully examined, giving a well-rounded approach to cancer-fighting nutrition.

Equally crucial are the foods to avoid, and This book does not shy away from describing the detrimental effects of processed and red meats, sugary beverages, and snacks, as well as meals high in salt and sodium. It emphasizes alcohol's negative impact on cancer therapy, as well as the dangers of artificial chemicals and preservatives.

Meal planning and preparation are important topics addressed in the book, with ideas for generating balanced meal plans and fast, simple dishes tailored to the unique requirements of lung cancer patients. This section is very useful and user-friendly since it includes tips for optimal meal preparation and storage, changing meals for side effects such as nausea and taste alterations, and integrating family and cultural preferences.

This book also discusses the significance of supplements and alternative treatments, offering a critical assessment of popular supplements and alternative nutritional regimens such as keto and vegan diets. It emphasizes the significance of contacting a healthcare physician before beginning any new food or supplement regimen to ensure safety and effectiveness.

Another important topic covered in this book is diet-based management of lung cancer side effects and therapy. It addresses typical difficulties such as nausea, vomiting, taste and smell alterations, appetite loss, diarrhea, constipation, and mouth sores, and provides realistic nutritional options to treat these symptoms.

Recognizing the emotional and psychological components of living with lung cancer, This book addresses how nutrition affects mental health. It discusses how to remain motivated, establish a supporting network, manage stress, and reap the advantages of mindful eating, all of which contribute to general well-being.

Physical exercise is another important component of the comprehensive approach recommended by the book. It discusses the advantages of exercise for lung cancer patients, the best sorts of physical activities, and how to integrate them into everyday life. This section's important themes include balancing exercise with rest and recuperation, as well as collaborating with physical therapists and trainers to improve physical health.

Finally, this book provides long-term nutritional guidelines for maintaining a healthy weight, avoiding cancer recurrence, and establishing lifetime good eating habits. It emphasizes the significance of seeing a nutritionist regularly and altering dietary habits as health requirements change to ensure lung cancer survivors' long-term well-being and quality of life.

INTRODUCTION

Lung cancer is a severe disease that affects millions of individuals globally. It may have a substantial influence on health, resulting in symptoms such as coughing, chest discomfort, and trouble breathing. Lung cancer treatment options include surgery, chemotherapy, radiation therapy, and targeted therapy. However, nutrition is also important in controlling the illness and promoting general health.

An Overview OF Lung Cancer AND Its Effect ON Health

Lung cancer occurs when abnormal cells in the lungs multiply excessively. The two primary forms are non-small cell lung cancer and small cell lung cancer. Although smoking is the major cause of lung cancer, additional factors such as exposure to secondhand smoke, air pollution, radon gas, and genetic predisposition may all contribute to its development.

Lung cancer may have serious consequences for one's health. It may cause serious health symptoms such as chronic coughing, chest discomfort, shortness of breath, and accidental weight loss. Lung cancer may also have an impact on mental and emotional health, producing anxiety, despair, and stress in both patients and loved ones.

Importance Of Diet In Managing Lung Cancer

Diet plays an important part in lung cancer management because it provides necessary nutrients that maintain general health, improve the immune system, and help the body tolerate cancer therapies. A well-balanced diet may also assist lung cancer patients avoid problems and enhance their quality of life.

A balanced diet may help you maintain your strength and energy levels, which are important for dealing with the physical demands of lung cancer therapy. It may also help the body mend and recuperate after surgery, chemotherapy, and radiation treatment. Furthermore, many foods and minerals may include anti-cancer characteristics that may help inhibit the development of cancer cells and decrease inflammation in the body.

Lung Cancer Diet Goals

The main aims of a lung cancer diet are:

1. **Support General Health:** A lung cancer diet is designed to supply the body with the nutrients it needs to preserve strength, vitality, and general well-being.

2. **Manage Symptoms and Side Effects:** Certain foods and dietary methods may help reduce typical symptoms and side effects of lung cancer and its treatments, such as nausea, vomiting, exhaustion, and lack of appetite.

3. **Optimise Treatment results:** A nutritious diet may help the body tolerate cancer therapies better and may

even increase their efficacy, resulting in improved treatment results and a higher quality of life.

4. Reduce the Risk of problems: A well-balanced diet helps lower the risk of problems during and after lung cancer treatment, such as infections, malnutrition, and muscle loss.

Basic Nutritional Principles For Cancer Patients

When it comes to diet for lung cancer patients, a few fundamental guidelines should be followed:

1. Eat a Variety of Nutrient-Rich Foods: Include a variety of nutrient-dense foods in your diet, such as fruits, vegetables, whole grains, lean meats, and healthy fats.

2. Remind Hydrated: Drink lots of fluids, including water, herbal teas, and clear broths, to remain hydrated and avoid dehydration, particularly if you're having side effects like vomiting or diarrhea.

3. **Maintain a Healthy Weight:** Eat a well-balanced diet and exercise regularly to maintain a healthy weight. Excessive weight loss or gain should be avoided since it might affect treatment results and general health.

4. **Manage Side Effects:** Modify your diet to address frequent side effects of lung cancer and its therapies, such as nausea, vomiting, diarrhea, constipation, and taste changes. Experiment with small, frequent meals, bland foods, and nutritional supplements as required.

5. **Consult a Registered Dietitian:** Work with a registered dietitian who specializes in cancer to create a personalized nutrition plan that is tailored to your unique requirements and interests. They may advise on meal planning, food selection, and managing particular dietary difficulties associated with lung cancer and its therapies.

How to Use This Book Effectively

This book is intended to give practical advice and techniques for adopting good eating habits into your daily routine while treating lung cancer. Each section contains useful information on nutrition, meal planning, and dietary practices to help you maintain your health and well-being during and after treatment.

To utilize this book efficiently, consider the following suggestions:

1. **Study Each Section Carefully:** Take the time to study each section thoroughly to understand the role of nutrition in lung cancer management and how it might affect your health and treatment results.

2. **Apply the advice:** Put the dietary advice and practices discussed in each section into practice in your everyday life. Experiment with various meals, recipes, and meal plans to see what works best for you.

3. Seek Help: Don't be afraid to seek assistance from healthcare experts such as oncologists, nurses, and registered dietitians, who can give personalized counsel and support based on your specific requirements and circumstances.

4. Maintaining a good attitude and being motivated may make a big difference in your battle with lung cancer. Focus on making tiny, manageable improvements to your food and lifestyle that will benefit your overall health and well-being.

By adopting the knowledge and ideas in this book into your daily routine, you may take proactive actions to successfully manage your lung cancer and enhance your overall quality of life.

CHAPTER ONE

Understanding Lung Cancer

Types And Stages Of Lung Cancer

Types of Lung Cancer

Lung cancer is widely classified into two types: non-small cell lung cancer (NSCLC) and small cell lung cancer (SCLC). Non-small cell lung cancer is the most frequent kind, accounting for around 85% of all occurrences, with small cell lung cancer making up the remaining 15%.

Non-small cell lung cancer has many subtypes, including adenocarcinoma, squamous cell carcinoma, and large cell carcinoma. These subgroups have unique features and may need alternative treatment options.

Stages of Lung Cancer

Lung cancer is classified according to the size of the tumor, whether it has progressed to neighboring lymph nodes, and if it has metastasized to other areas of the body. The phases are numbered from 0 to IV, with 0 being the earliest and IV being the most advanced.

• Stage 0: Also known as carcinoma in situ, cancer cells are only seen in the innermost lining of the lung and have not spread to deeper tissues.

• Stage I: Cancer is limited to the lung and has not spread to adjacent lymph nodes.

• At Stage II, cancer may have spread to adjacent lymph nodes or structures.

• In Stage III, cancer has progressed to lymph nodes in the chest and surrounding tissues.

• Stage IV cancer involves metastasis to distant organs such as the brain, liver, and bones.

Understanding the kind and stage of lung cancer is critical for identifying the best treatment option.

Common Symptoms And Diagnostic Methods

Symptoms Of Lung Cancer

Early-stage lung cancer may not produce visible symptoms; nevertheless, as the illness advances, typical symptoms may include:

- Persistent cough.

- Chest ache.

- Shortness of breath.

- Unexpected weight loss

- Fatigue.

- Hoarseness.

- Coughing up blood.

It's crucial to remember that these symptoms may also be caused by other ailments, so see a doctor for an accurate examination and diagnosis.

Diagnosis Methods:

Several tests might be performed to identify lung cancer, including:

• Imaging tests such as X-rays, CT scans, and MRIs may offer comprehensive pictures of the lungs and identify abnormalities.

• Biopsy: A tissue sample is obtained from the lung using a needle, bronchoscopy, or surgical biopsy to confirm cancer cells and define the kind of malignancy.

• Sputum cytology involves examining mucus coughed up from the lungs for cancer cells using a microscope.

Early identification of lung cancer significantly improves treatment results, so those who have symptoms or are at high risk should have frequent screenings.

Treatment Alternatives And Side Effects

Treatment Options:

The kind and stage of lung cancer, as well as the individual's general health and preferences, all influence treatment decisions. Common treatments include:

• Early-stage lung cancer may need surgery to remove the tumor and surrounding tissue.

• Chemotherapy involves using powerful medications to destroy or prevent cancer cells from developing.

• Radiation treatment uses high-energy beams to eliminate malignant cells.

• Targeted treatment inhibits cancer cell proliferation by targeting certain defects.

• Immunotherapy: Drugs activate the body's immune system to target cancer cells.

Side Effects

While these medicines may be beneficial in combating cancer, they may also have negative effects. The following are some common adverse effects of lung cancer treatment:

• Nausea and vomiting.

• Fatigue.

• Hair loss.

• Loss of appetite.

• Mouth sores.

• Skin changes.

• High vulnerability to infections.

Patients should talk freely with their healthcare provider about any adverse effects they are experiencing since there are frequent methods to control or mitigate them.

The Role Of Nutrition In Cancer Care

Importance of Nutrition

Maintaining a healthy diet is critical for cancer patients. A well-balanced diet may help:

• Improve general health and immunological function.

• Maintain strength and energy levels.

• Promote bodily recovery and healing.

• Manage treatment-related adverse effects.

• Improve quality of life.

Nutritional recommendations

While there is no special "lung cancer diet," there are broad principles that patients with lung cancer should follow to maintain appropriate nutrition:

- Eat a mix of fruits, vegetables, whole grains, and lean meats to meet nutritional requirements.

- To stay hydrated, consume lots of fluids like water, herbal tea, or clear broths.

- Limit processed, sugary, and high-fat foods that may cause inflammation and other health difficulties.

- If therapy affects appetite, consider eating smaller, more frequent meals.

- Seek a trained dietitian for personalized nutritional advice and assistance.

Individuals with lung cancer who pay attention to diet may better deal with treatment problems and enhance their general well-being.

Myths And Facts On Lung Cancer And Diet

Myth: Sugar Fuels Cancer Cells.

It is a frequent myth that eating sugar stimulates the development of cancer cells. While it is true that cancer cells need glucose (sugar) for energy, eliminating sugar is neither required nor advantageous. The body requires glucose for a variety of vital processes, and eliminating it might result in nutritional deficits and other health concerns.

Fact: Balanced nutrition is key.

Instead of concentrating on avoiding certain foods or minerals, the emphasis should be on eating a well-balanced diet rich in important nutrients to promote general health and well-being. This involves eating a variety of meals from each food category and keeping hydrated.

Myth: Alternative treatments can cure cancer.

Some alternative medicines and dietary supplements claim to cure or treat cancer, however, there is often insufficient scientific evidence to back these claims. Such therapies should be approached with caution and discussed with a healthcare expert before adding them to a treatment plan.

Fact: Complementary Approaches Can Help Treat

While alternative treatments cannot replace conventional cancer treatment, certain complementary methods, such as acupuncture, massage therapy, and mind-body practices, may help control symptoms and improve the quality of life for people with lung cancer. Any alternative treatments should be discussed with a healthcare team to confirm their safety and appropriateness.

CHAPTER TWO

Nutritional Needs Of Lung Cancer Patients

Macronutrients Include Proteins, Carbohydrates, And Fats

Proteins, carbs, and lipids are the three basic macronutrients required for good health, particularly among lung cancer patients. Proteins are essential for tissue regeneration and immune system support, which are especially important during cancer therapy. Carbohydrates give energy, while lipids regulate hormone synthesis and nutrition absorption.

Lung cancer patients must consume enough amounts of these macronutrients. Lean protein foods, such as chicken, fish, tofu, and beans, may help you achieve your protein requirements without consuming too much fat.

Carbohydrates from nutritious grains, fruits, and vegetables give a steady supply of energy, which helps to battle the weariness that sometimes occurs following cancer treatments. Avocados, nuts, seeds, and olive oil provide healthy fats, which promote general health and may help decrease inflammation.

Balancing these macronutrients in each meal may help the body meet its nutritional requirements throughout therapy. An example dinner for a lung cancer patient would consist of grilled chicken (protein), quinoa (carbohydrates), and steamed veggies drizzled with olive oil (good fats), providing a well-rounded nutritional profile to promote overall health and well-being.

Micronutrients Include Vitamins And Minerals

Micronutrients, such as vitamins and minerals, are essential for lung cancer patients' immune systems and general health. Vitamins C, E, and D are antioxidants that may assist the body in minimizing oxidative stress and inflammation. Minerals such as zinc and selenium are necessary for immunological function and may aid the body's defense against illness.

For lung cancer patients, it is critical to provide enough micronutrient consumption via a balanced diet rich in fruits, vegetables, whole grains, and lean meats. Incorporating a variety of colorful fruits and vegetables into meals provides a wide range of vitamins and minerals. Oranges and strawberries, for example, have high levels of vitamin C, but nuts and seeds are high in vitamin E.

Supplementation may also be required in certain circumstances, particularly if specific vitamin levels are insufficient. However, it is critical to contact a healthcare expert before beginning any supplements, since excessive use of certain vitamins and minerals may be dangerous, particularly during cancer treatment.

Importance Of Hydration

Staying hydrated is essential for lung cancer patients, particularly during therapy. Proper hydration helps to maintain regular body functioning, assists digestion, and promotes kidney health. Dehydration may increase common cancer-related side symptoms including tiredness, nausea, and diarrhea.

Encourage proper fluid intake with water, herbal teas, and clear broths to help avoid dehydration. It is critical to check urine color; light yellow pee suggests appropriate hydration, but dark yellow urine may indicate dehydration.

Sipping fluids throughout the day, rather than drinking big quantities all at once, might help minimize nausea and discomfort, particularly for individuals suffering treatment-related side effects. Also, limiting caffeinated and sugary drinks might help prevent additional dehydration.

Caloric Needs And Energy Balance

Understanding caloric demands and establishing energy balance is critical for lung cancer patients since maintaining a healthy weight may improve overall health and treatment results. Caloric requirements might vary according to age, gender, weight, exercise level, and cancer stage.

During therapy, patients may suffer hunger changes, taste changes, and difficulties swallowing, all of which may have an impact on calorie intake. In such instances, concentrating on nutrient-dense meals that give necessary calories and minerals is critical. Smoothies, soups, and protein-packed snacks such as Greek yogurt or nut butter are also nutritious alternatives.

Regular weight monitoring, as well as consultation with a healthcare physician or qualified dietitian, may assist ensure that caloric requirements are fulfilled.

Adjustments may be required due to therapy adverse effects, changes in appetite, or weight fluctuations.

Adjusting Nutritional Needs During Treatment

Adapting dietary demands throughout lung cancer therapy is critical for supporting the body's recovery and minimizing treatment-induced negative effects. Chemotherapy, radiation treatment, and surgery may all affect appetite, digestion, and nutritional absorption, necessitating adjustments to dietary choices.

For example, people receiving chemotherapy may feel nausea, vomiting, or mouth sores, making it difficult to eat regularly. In such circumstances, eating small, frequent meals and selecting bland, readily digested foods might help alleviate discomfort.

Radiation treatment may induce changes in taste perception and difficulties swallowing, necessitating alterations such as adding more spices or pureeing meals to make them easier to swallow. Surgery may involve temporary food restrictions or alterations to improve recovery and avoid problems.

Working closely with a healthcare team, which includes oncologists, nurses, and dietitians, may assist ensure that nutritional requirements are satisfied throughout treatment. Adjustments may be required depending on individual symptoms, treatment responses, and general health conditions, emphasizing the significance of personalized nutrition care for lung cancer patients.

CHAPTER THREE

High-Protein Foods For Muscle Maintenance

Maintaining muscle mass is critical for lung cancer patients because it improves overall strength and resilience. Including high-protein meals in your diet may help with muscle maintenance and repair. Lean protein sources include chicken, fish, eggs, tofu, lentils, and low-fat dairy products. These foods include the essential amino acids required for muscular health.

When including high-protein foods in your meals, look for a diverse range of sources throughout the day. For example, begin your day with eggs or Greek yogurt for breakfast, then have grilled chicken or fish for lunch and beans or lentils for supper. Snacks like nuts, seeds, and protein bars may also help you get more protein in between meals.

Fruits And Vegetables With High Antioxidant Levels

Antioxidants have an important role in reducing oxidative stress and inflammation in the body, which may be useful for people with lung cancer. Fruits and vegetables include high levels of antioxidants, vitamins, and minerals, which promote general health and well-being. Berries like blueberries, strawberries, and raspberries are especially high in antioxidants including vitamin C and flavonoids.

Leafy greens like spinach, kale, and broccoli include antioxidants including vitamin E and beta-carotene. Including a variety of colorful fruits and vegetables in your diet guarantees that you obtain a wide range of antioxidants to help your immune system and lower your risk of chronic illnesses.

Whole Grains And Their Benefits

Whole grains are an important part of a lung cancer diet because of their high fiber content and nutritional richness. Unlike processed grains, whole grains maintain all portions of the grain kernel, including the bran, germ, and endosperm, which include critical elements such as fiber, vitamins, and minerals.

Whole grains, such as brown rice, quinoa, oats, barley, and whole wheat, may help control blood sugar levels, support digestive health, and lower the risk of cardiovascular disease. These grains may be consumed in a variety of ways, including as a side dish, salads, soups, and breakfast options such as muesli or whole grain toast.

Healthy Fats: Their Sources

While it is important to avoid saturated and trans fats in your diet, including good fats may give several health advantages, particularly for those who have lung cancer. Avocados, almonds, seeds, olive oil, and fatty fish such as salmon and mackerel are also good sources of healthful fat.

Healthy fats help to reduce inflammation, improve brain function, and absorb fat-soluble vitamins such as vitamin E and vitamin D. A reasonable quantity of healthy fats in your meals will help you feel full and give you long-lasting energy throughout the day.

Hydrating Foods And Beverages

Staying hydrated is critical for general health and well-being, particularly for those receiving cancer treatments. While drinking water is essential, you may also improve your hydration by ingesting hydrating foods and drinks.

Fruits like watermelon, strawberries, oranges, and cucumbers are rich in water and may help you stay hydrated all day. Herbal teas, coconut water, and homemade soups are all great ways to remain hydrated while adding flavor and minerals to your diet.

By including these hydrating meals and drinks into your daily routine, you may maintain adequate hydration and enhance overall health and well-being throughout your lung cancer treatment.

CHAPTER FOUR

Foods To Avoid

Processed And Red Meats

When it comes to controlling lung cancer with food, one of the most important concerns is limiting your consumption of processed and red meat. These meats are often heavy in saturated fats and may include dangerous chemicals such as nitrates, which have been linked to an increased risk of cancer. Processed meats like bacon, sausage, and deli meats are rich in salt, which may lead to high blood pressure and other health problems.

Instead of processed and red meats, try to include lean proteins in your diet. This may include chicken, turkey, and seafood such as salmon and tuna. These selections have critical nutrients without the saturated fats and chemicals found in processed meats.

Incorporating plant-based protein sources such as beans, lentils, and tofu may also be a healthy alternative to meat while satisfying your protein requirements.

Sugary Beverages And Snacks

Another crucial part of a lung cancer diet is to limit your use of sugary beverages and snacks. Foods and drinks heavy in added sugars may cause weight gain and inflammation, exacerbating the negative effects of cancer therapy and lowering overall health.

Instead of opting for sugary beverages like soda or fruit juice, try water, herbal teas, or infused water with fruit slices for flavor. These solutions will keep you hydrated without any additional sweets. When it comes to snacking, choose whole foods such as fresh fruits, vegetables, nuts, and seeds, which provide minerals and fiber without the additional sugars and empty calories found in processed snacks.

Excessive Salt And Sodium-Rich Foods

Another significant factor to consider while treating lung cancer is reducing salt and sodium consumption. High sodium levels may cause high blood pressure and fluid retention, exacerbating some symptoms and adverse effects of therapy.

Limit your intake of salty snacks, processed meals, and canned items, since they are generally rich in sodium. Instead, prepare fresh dishes at home using herbs, spices, and other flavorings to increase taste without needing salt. Furthermore, selecting fresh fruits and vegetables over canned types will help you consume less salt while still delivering critical nutrients and antioxidants.

Alcohol And Its Effects On Therapy

Alcohol intake may hurt cancer therapy and general health. Alcohol use may impair treatment efficacy and raise the risk of complications in people with lung cancer.

It is critical to minimize or avoid alcohol when receiving cancer therapy. Alcohol may suppress the immune system and impair the body's capacity to heal and recover. Additionally, drinking alcohol has been related to an increased risk of some forms of cancer, including lung cancer. For a refreshing alternative to alcohol, try sparkling water mixed with fruit juice or herbal teas.

Artificial Additives And Preservatives

When controlling lung cancer via nutrition, it is important to be aware of any artificial additives and preservatives that may be present in processed foods.

Artificial colors, flavors, and preservatives are examples of additives that may be harmful to one's health and increase inflammation.

To limit your exposure to artificial additives and preservatives, eat full, unadulterated foods whenever feasible. This contains fresh fruits and vegetables, entire grains, lean meats, and good fats. When buying packaged goods, carefully study the ingredient labels and choose those with few additives and preservatives. Consider including organic foods in your diet, since they are less likely to contain artificial chemicals and pesticides. You may improve your general health and well-being while managing lung cancer by focusing on whole foods and limiting your intake of processed foods.

CHAPTER FIVE

Menu Planning And Preparation

Creating Balanced Meal Plans

Creating balanced meal planning is critical for people with lung cancer to ensure they get enough nourishment to maintain their health and wellness. A well-balanced meal plan comprises items from many dietary categories to give critical elements including vitamins, minerals, protein, carbs, and healthy fats.

When preparing meals, be sure to include a mix of fruits, vegetables, whole grains, lean meats, and healthy fats. To receive the most vitamins, minerals, and antioxidants, eat a variety of fruits and vegetables. Include leafy greens like spinach and kale, colorful bell peppers, berries, citrus fruits, and cruciferous veggies like broccoli and cauliflower.

In addition to fruits and vegetables, whole grains such as brown rice, quinoa, oats, and whole wheat products include fiber, which improves digestion and keeps blood sugar levels constant. Lean proteins including chicken, fish, tofu, beans, lentils, and eggs are essential for muscle maintenance and regeneration, particularly during cancer therapy.

Incorporating healthy fats like avocados, nuts, seeds, and olive oil is also beneficial to general health. Healthy fats provide energy, promote cell development, and aid in the absorption of fat-soluble vitamins such as vitamins A, D, E, and K.

Quick & Easy Recipes

When coping with the obstacles of lung cancer treatment, it's reasonable that people may lack the energy or drive to prepare lavish meals. Quick and quick dishes may be a lifesaver during these times, offering nutritious meals without needing much time or effort in the kitchen.

Vegetable stir-fry is a simple yet healthful meal. Begin by sautéing your favorite colorful veggies, such as bell peppers, broccoli, carrots, snap peas, and mushrooms, in a little olive oil. For a filling supper, add some cooked protein, such as chopped chicken breast or tofu, and season with herbs and spices like garlic, ginger, and soy sauce. Serve over brown rice or quinoa.

Another simple alternative is a nutrient-packed smoothie. Simply combine a variety of fruits, such as bananas, berries, spinach, and Greek yogurt or almond milk, for protein and smoothness. To add even more protein, mix with a scoop of protein powder or a spoonful of nut butter.

Tips For Meal Prep And Storage

Meal preparation may be a game changer for people with lung cancer because it provides easy access to nutritious meals throughout the week, minimizing the need for frequent cooking and decision-making when energy levels are low. Here are some recommendations for efficient meal preparation and storage:

1. **Plan Ahead:** Set aside time at the beginning of the week to plan your meals and create a shopping list. This will help you keep organized and ensure you have all of the necessary components on hand.

2. Batch cooking is preparing huge quantities of food that may be portioned and stored for later use. Soups, stews, casseroles, and grain-based salads are ideal for batch cooking.

3. **Use Freezer-Friendly Containers:** Purchase freezer-friendly containers to keep prepared meals in the

freezer for a longer shelf life. Label containers with the date and contents to facilitate identification.

4. Preparing Ingredients in Advance: To make dinner preparation easier throughout the week, wash, cut, and portion fruits, vegetables, and meats ahead of time. Refrigerate prepared items in sealed containers for convenient access.

5. Consider Convenience Foods: While whole foods are preferable, it is OK to include convenience foods such as pre-cut veggies, canned beans, and frozen fruits and vegetables to save time and energy.

Adjusting Meals For Side Effects

During lung cancer therapy, people may suffer nausea, taste changes, and trouble swallowing, which may impair their ability to consume and enjoy food. Meals must be adjusted to accommodate these negative effects while still providing appropriate nourishment.

For nausea, eat bland, easily digestible meals such as crackers, bread, rice, and bananas. Avoid strong-smelling or fatty foods, and eat small, regular meals throughout the day rather than big ones.

If taste changes are impacting your appetite and pleasure of meals, try various flavors and textures to see what works best. To increase flavor, try adding herbs, spices, citrus, or sweets, and choose meals with strong, enticing flavors.

For those who have trouble swallowing, pick soft or pureed meals that are easier to chew and swallow, such as smoothies, soups, mashed potatoes, yogurt, and oats. Avoid dry or gritty meals that might be difficult to swallow.

Incorporating Family And Cultural Preferences

Incorporating family and cultural preferences into meal preparation may make the process more pleasurable and meaningful for all parties.

When preparing meals, consider family members' tastes and dietary restrictions, and include them in the decision-making process to ensure that everyone's requirements are satisfied.

If specific ethnic cuisines are important to your family, discover methods to include them in a balanced meal plan. Look for healthier variations of classic recipes or adjust the ingredients to decrease added sugars, salt, and harmful fats while retaining the flavors and textures you like.

Cooking together as a family can be a bonding activity, allowing you to share traditions, stories, and experiences while making and eating meals together. Encourage family members to help with dinner preparation, whether it's slicing vegetables, setting the table, or cleaning dishes, to alleviate the workload and promote a feeling of community and connection.

By implementing these techniques and methods into your meal planning and preparation routine, you can make the process easier and guarantee that you're delivering nutritional meals that will benefit your health and well-being throughout lung cancer treatment. Remember to listen to your body, respect your wishes, and seek assistance from loved ones and healthcare experts as required.

CHAPTER SIX

Supplements And Alternative Therapies

Role Of Dietary Supplements

Dietary supplements play an important part in the treatment of lung cancer by delivering critical nutrients that may be deficient owing to a variety of causes such as reduced appetite, medication side effects, or nutrient malabsorption. These vitamins may enhance general health, stimulate the immune system, and increase energy levels throughout cancer treatment.

Dietary supplements play an important part in lung cancer care by ensuring an appropriate intake of vitamins, minerals, and antioxidants. These nutrients are essential for maintaining appropriate cellular function, boosting immunological function, and guarding against oxidative stress, which is especially critical for cancer patients under treatment.

Supplements may also assist with certain nutritional shortages that may occur during cancer therapy. For example, some individuals may have low vitamin D levels owing to insufficient sun exposure or inadequate gastrointestinal absorption. In such circumstances, vitamin D tablets may help preserve bone health and immunological function.

Furthermore, certain supplements may have anti-inflammatory or anti-cancer characteristics that may enhance traditional cancer therapies. For example, omega-3 fatty acids contained in fish oil supplements have been demonstrated to have anti-inflammatory properties, which may aid in the reduction of inflammation and improve treatment results for lung cancer patients.

However, it is important to highlight that supplements should not be utilized instead of a well-balanced diet or regular cancer therapies. They should be seen as a complementary treatment that may improve general health and aid in the body's natural healing processes.

Popular Supplements For Cancer Patients

Several supplements are routinely taken by lung cancer patients to meet their nutritional demands and improve their overall health throughout treatment. Some of the most popular supplements are:

1. Multivitamin supplements are a mix of key vitamins and minerals that may help cover dietary deficiencies in the diet and promote overall health.

2. Protein Supplements: Protein is necessary for preserving muscle mass and strength throughout cancer therapy. Protein supplements, such as whey protein or plant-based protein powders, may help patients achieve their protein requirements when

their appetite is poor or their food intake is insufficient.

3.Omega-3 Fatty Acids: Fish oil supplements and flaxseed oil include omega-3 fatty acids, which have anti-inflammatory qualities and may help decrease inflammation, boost immunological function, and promote heart health.

4. Probiotics: These supplements include helpful bacteria that may help maintain a healthy gut microbiota, which is necessary for good digestion, nutrient absorption, and immunological function. They may also assist with gastrointestinal side effects after cancer therapy, such as diarrhea or constipation.

5. Herbal Supplements: Certain herbs and botanicals, such as turmeric, green tea extract, and medicinal mushrooms, have been investigated for their anti-cancer qualities. These supplements may contain antioxidant, anti-inflammatory, or immune-boosting

properties, which may improve general health and well-being during cancer treatment.

Assessing The Safety And Efficacy Of Supplements

When evaluating dietary supplements to treat lung cancer, it is critical to assess their safety and effectiveness. Not all supplements are created equal, and some may interfere with cancer therapies or drugs, posing hazards to some people.

One of the first stages in determining the safety of supplements is to speak with a healthcare physician or registered dietitian who is familiar with cancer treatment. They can advise you on which supplements are most suited to your specific requirements, medical history, and treatment plan.

It is also critical to investigate the scientific data supporting the usage of certain supplements for lung cancer treatment.

Seek credible sources of information, such as peer-reviewed research papers or guidance from professional organizations like the American Cancer Society or the National Institutes of Health.

When evaluating the effectiveness of supplements, examine the quality of the research studies, the consistency of findings across different studies, and any possible hazards or side effects of the supplement. Keep in mind that, although certain supplements may offer promising early data, additional study is often required to validate their efficacy for lung cancer patients particularly.

In addition to talking with healthcare practitioners and studying scientific data, consider the quality and safety of the supplements themselves. Choose supplements from reputed producers that follow good manufacturing practices (GMP) and have been third-party tested for purity and efficacy.

Alternative Diets And Therapies

In addition to dietary supplements, some lung cancer patients may consider alternate diets and treatments as part of their cancer treatment strategy. These techniques might include:

1. **Ketogenic Diet:** The ketogenic diet is a high-fat, low-carbohydrate eating regimen that has gained popularity due to its possible anti-cancer properties. Some studies show that ketosis, a metabolic condition caused by the diet, may decrease cancer cell proliferation and enhance treatment results. However, further research is required to properly understand the ketogenic diet's involvement in lung cancer care.

2. **Vegan Diet:** A vegan diet is free of animal products and high in fruits, vegetables, whole grains, and plant-based protein. Some studies show that vegan diets may protect against some forms of cancer, but more

study is required to evaluate the influence on lung cancer in particular.

3. Acupuncture is a traditional Chinese medical method in which small needles are inserted into particular places on the body to promote healing and relieve symptoms. Some lung cancer patients may utilize acupuncture to alleviate discomfort, nausea, exhaustion, or other treatment-related adverse effects.

4. **Mind-Body Therapies:** Mind-body therapies including yoga, meditation, and tai chi may assist lung cancer patients decrease stress, increase quality of life, and improve their general well-being. These activities may also help with traditional cancer therapies by increasing calm, lowering anxiety, and boosting emotional resilience.

Before beginning any alternative diet or therapy, consult with a healthcare expert to confirm that it is safe and suitable for your specific requirements and treatment plan. While certain alternative therapies may assist specific individuals, they should be used in combination with established cancer treatments rather than as a substitute.

Consulting With Healthcare Providers

Before beginning a new regimen of dietary supplements, alternative diets, or treatments for lung cancer management, contact healthcare specialists who are knowledgeable about your medical history and treatment plan. They may provide personalized advice and suggestions based on your specific requirements and interests.

Oncologists, registered dietitians, nurses, and other experts may be part of your healthcare team and may provide guidance and support during your cancer treatment. They can guide you through the complicated terrain of nutritional supplements and alternative treatments, analyze the safety and effectiveness of various techniques, and successfully incorporate them into your entire treatment plan.

During discussions with healthcare experts, be sure to ask questions, voice any concerns or preferences you may have, and talk about the possible risks and advantages of different alternatives. Together, you may create a complete and personalized strategy for lung cancer care that fits your specific requirements and objectives while putting your safety and well-being first.

Working closely with your healthcare team and adopting a proactive approach to managing your health may help you achieve better treatment results, improve your quality of life, and empower yourself to make educated choices about your care. Remember that you are not alone in your fight against lung cancer, and there are tools and assistance available to assist you every step of the way.

CHAPTER SEVEN

Managing Side Effects Via Diet

Addressing Nausea And Vomiting

Nausea and vomiting are unpleasant side effects of lung cancer therapy, but there are dietary choices that might help alleviate these symptoms. Then begin, modest, frequent meals are preferable to big ones, since overeating may increase nausea. Choosing bland, easy-to-digest items like crackers, bread, rice, or bananas may frequently help soothe the stomach. Avoiding oily, spicy, or too-rich meals is recommended since they might cause nausea.

Ginger has long been used as a natural cure for nausea, whether in the form of ginger tea, ginger ale, or ginger candies, and it may be especially beneficial for cancer patients suffering from this condition. Peppermint tea and peppermint candies may also bring comfort. Staying hydrated is crucial, so drinking clear fluids like water, herbal teas, or electrolyte drinks throughout the day will help avoid dehydration and nausea.

For individuals who continue to vomit, it is critical to restore lost fluids and electrolytes. Oral rehydration medications and liquids designed to replenish electrolytes may be effective. Furthermore, avoiding strongly scented or pungent meals might help lessen the chance of vomiting episodes.

Coping With Taste And Smell Changes

Changes in taste and smell are frequent after lung cancer therapy and may have a substantial influence on appetite and pleasure of meals. To fight these changes, experimenting with new flavors and textures might be beneficial. Adding herbs, spices, or citrus juices to meals may improve their flavor without using too much salt or sugar, which may be less appetizing at this time.

It's also vital to concentrate on meals with strong flavors or textures that can be enjoyed despite altered taste sensations. Sour meals, such as lemon or vinegar, or foods with a crunchy texture, such as raw vegetables or nuts, might help to cut through flavor alterations and bring enjoyment.

Another option is to try chilled or frozen meals, since they may have milder flavors and scents, making them more appealing. Smoothies, popsicles, and frozen grapes are all delicious alternatives that are simpler to digest.

Strategies To Manage Appetite Loss

Loss of appetite is a typical side effect of lung cancer and its treatment, but there are strategies to stimulate eating and stay nourished. One strategy is to concentrate on nutrient-dense foods, which provide a lot of calories and nutrients in modest quantities. Nuts, seeds, nut butter, avocados, cheese, and dried fruit are some examples.

It might also be beneficial to eat small, regular meals and snacks throughout the day rather than attempting to consume huge servings at mealtime. Keeping food easily accessible and simple to get may promote grazing and prevent hunger from becoming overpowering.

Experimenting with various food combinations and meal times may also help increase appetite. Some individuals find that they have a stronger appetite in the morning or at certain times of the day, so altering meal timings appropriately may be useful.

Dealing With Diarrhoea And Constipation

Diarrhea and constipation are two typical gastrointestinal side effects of lung cancer therapy, however, dietary changes might assist with these symptoms. High-fiber meals, dairy products, spicy foods, and caffeine should all be avoided if you have diarrhea. Instead, choose bland, low-fiber options such as white rice, bananas, applesauce, and boiled potatoes.

Maintaining hydration is critical for both diarrhea and constipation. Drinking enough fluids, particularly water, may assist control of bowel motions and avoid dehydration. In addition to water, clear broths, herbal teas, and electrolyte drinks may help with hydration.

Consuming more fiber from fruits, vegetables, whole grains, and legumes may assist with constipation. Prunes, prune juice, and other dried fruits are excellent natural cures for constipation. It is critical to add fiber gradually to prevent worsening symptoms.

Foods That May Help With Mouth Sores And Difficulty Swallowing

Patients with lung cancer may struggle to eat due to mouth sores and trouble swallowing, known as dysphagia. Choosing soft, easy-to-swallow meals may help relieve pain and provide appropriate nourishment. Yogurt, mashed potatoes, smoothies, and soups might be simpler to digest than hard or brittle meals.

Avoiding acidic or spicy meals that might cause mouth sores is critical. Choose mild, neutral-flavored meals instead. Drinking cold or lukewarm beverages may also help relieve sore throats and make swallowing easier.

In certain circumstances, changing the texture of food might make it easier to swallow. Pureeing or mixing meals into smooth textures might aid with swallowing problems.

Adding moisture to dishes via sauces, gravies, or broth may also make them easier to swallow.

Managing side effects via nutrition is an important element of assisting lung cancer patients throughout treatment. Patients who treat symptoms such as nausea, taste changes, appetite loss, gastrointestinal difficulties, and trouble swallowing may maintain enough nutrition and enhance their overall quality of life. Experimenting with new foods, textures, and tactics may help people figure out what works best for them and make eating more pleasurable at a stressful time.

CHAPTER EIGHT

Emotional And Psychological Support

Effects Of Diet On Mental Health

Diet has a significant impact on mental health, particularly for those with lung cancer. The foods we eat have a direct influence on our mood, energy level, and general well-being. A nutrient-dense diet may help decrease typical cancer-related symptoms such as despair, anxiety, and stress.

Certain foods, such as fruits, vegetables, whole grains, and lean meats, provide vitamins, minerals, and antioxidants that promote brain health and mood regulation. Processed meals, sugary snacks, and too much coffee, on the other hand, may aggravate anxiety and exhaustion.

Maintaining a healthy diet may also improve cognitive function, allowing for improved decision-making and coping methods during difficult situations. By nourishing your body with the correct nutrients, you give it the resources it needs to deal with the physical and mental toll of cancer therapy.

Strategies To Stay Motivated

Staying motivated to consume a nutritious diet during lung cancer treatment might be difficult, but it is critical for overall well-being. Setting achievable objectives and celebrating minor triumphs along the way is an excellent method. Instead of concentrating on major changes, strive for incremental improvements in your eating patterns.

It's also useful to find inspiration in the reasons for your dietary modifications. Reminding yourself of your objectives, whether they be to boost your energy, strengthen your immune system, or improve your quality of life, will help you remain on track when confronted with temptation.

Furthermore, surround oneself with good influences, such as supportive friends and family members, to give encouragement and accountability. Sharing your experience with people who understand and empathize with your difficulties will help make the process less intimidating.

Creating A Support Network

Developing a support network is critical for overcoming the emotional and psychological obstacles of lung cancer therapy. Surrounding yourself with people who inspire and encourage you may give you a sense of belonging while also reducing feelings of loneliness.

Contact your friends, family, support groups, or online forums to connect with people who are going through similar situations.

Sharing your feelings, worries, and accomplishments with those who understand may provide comfort and encouragement during challenging times.

Don't be afraid to ask your support network for practical help, whether it's making meals, doing errands, or just listening with empathy. Knowing that you are not alone in your path may significantly improve your mental well-being.

Stress Management Techniques

Managing stress is critical for preserving both mental and physical health throughout lung cancer treatment. Chronic stress may impair the immune system, promote inflammation, and worsen depression and anxiety symptoms.

Incorporating stress management practices into your daily routine may assist in reducing these effects and foster a feeling of peace and relaxation. Deep breathing techniques, meditation, yoga, and gradual muscle relaxation are all effective ways to decrease stress and increase general well-being.

It is also important to recognize and prevent causes of excessive stress whenever feasible. Prioritise work, distribute duties and learn to say no to extra obligations that might overwhelm you. Remember to prioritize self-care and things that make you happy and relaxed.

Mindful Eating And Its Benefits

Mindful eating is a discipline that entails focusing on the sensory experience of eating while being completely present in the moment. This method may help you have a healthy connection with food, improve digestion, and avoid overeating.

Begin by paying attention to your body's hunger and fullness signs, then eat carefully and enjoy each meal. Concentrate on the flavor, texture, and scent of your food, and try to avoid distractions like television or technological gadgets during meals.

Mindful eating may also help you identify emotional eating triggers and create healthy coping methods. Instead of relying on food for comfort or stress reduction, consider writing, exercising, or speaking with a trusted friend or therapist.

By including mindful eating into your daily routine, you may develop a better appreciation for food while also nourishing your body and mind while you fight lung cancer.

CHAPTER NINE

Exercise And Physical Activity

Benefits Of Exercise For Lung Cancer Patients

Exercise is important for the overall health of lung cancer sufferers. While it may be paradoxical to participate in physical activity during therapy, exercise has various advantages that may dramatically enhance quality of life. Regular exercise may help reduce tiredness, improve mood, increase energy, and improve general physical function. It may also help treat symptoms including shortness of breath and muscular weakness.

Exercise may help lung cancer patients retain lung function and avoid problems like pneumonia and blood clots. Furthermore, physical exercise helps boost immunological function, which is essential for combating infections and assisting the body's healing process. Furthermore, exercise has been demonstrated to alleviate anxiety and sadness, which are major psychological issues for people living with cancer.

Types Of Suitable Physical Activities

When adding exercise to a lung cancer patient's regimen, it is critical to choose activities that are safe and suitable for their condition. Low-impact workouts like walking, swimming, cycling, and moderate yoga are ideal alternatives since they promote cardiovascular health and muscular strength without placing too much pressure on the joints. Stretching exercises may also help to maintain flexibility and reduce muscular strain.

It is critical to match the kind and intensity of physical exercise to the individual's capabilities and limits.

Patients with lung cancer should check with their healthcare provider before beginning any new fitness routine to verify that it is appropriate for their treatment plan and medical condition. In rare situations, patients may benefit from working with a skilled fitness trainer or physical therapist who can create a tailored exercise program based on their requirements and objectives.

Incorporating Exercise Into The Daily Routine

Adding exercise to a lung cancer patient's daily regimen does not have to be complex. Simple activities like short walks, moderate stretches, and deep breathing exercises may be readily incorporated into everyday life. Setting reasonable objectives and gradually increasing the time and intensity of exercise will help you develop endurance and avoid burnout.

Patients must listen to their bodies and pace themselves appropriately. Overexertion may cause weariness and increase symptoms, so it's important to maintain a balance between exercise and rest. Furthermore, selecting activities that are interesting and engaging might help patients continue their fitness program in the long run.

Balancing Activity, Rest, And Recovery

While exercise is helpful to lung cancer patients, it is critical to understand the value of rest and recuperation. Fatigue is a typical side effect of cancer therapy, and working too hard may result in tiredness and difficulties. Including rest times in your training regimen gives your body time to recuperate and replenish energy supplies.

Patients should prioritize getting enough sleep and listening to their bodies when they need to rest.

It's OK to cut down on exercising during times of high weariness or medication adverse effects. Patients who listen to their bodies and alter their activity levels appropriately may continue a long-term fitness habit that benefits their general health and well-being.

Working With Physical Therapists And Trainers

Working with physical therapists and skilled fitness trainers may be very beneficial to lung cancer patients. These specialists may evaluate the patient's current fitness level, identify areas of weakness or imbalance, and design a personalized training program to meet individual requirements and objectives.

Physical therapists may also advise you on appropriate techniques and forms to avoid injury and maximize the advantages of exercise. They may use a range of techniques, such as manual treatment, therapeutic exercise, and teaching on body mechanics and posture.

Certified fitness trainers with expertise in dealing with cancer patients may create safe and effective exercise programs based on the individual's skills and limits. They may give inspiration, accountability, and support along the process, allowing patients to remain on track and accomplish their fitness objectives.

Patients with lung cancer may improve their overall health and quality of life by incorporating exercise into their treatment and recovery plan safely and effectively, working with healthcare professionals and fitness experts.

CHAPTER TEN

Long-Term Dietary Strategies

Maintaining A Healthy Weight

Maintaining a healthy weight is critical for those diagnosed with lung cancer. Excess weight may worsen health problems and raise the chance of cancer recurrence. To acquire and maintain a healthy weight, eat a well-balanced diet rich in nutrients. Consuming enough fruits, vegetables, lean meats, and whole grains will help you feel satiated while also supplying critical nutrients for general health.

Weight management relies heavily on portion control. It is critical to limit portion sizes and prevent overeating, particularly when it comes to calorie-dense items like sweets and fried dishes. Instead, eat smaller, more frequent meals to help control hunger and avoid overindulgence.

Regular physical exercise is another important aspect of weight control. Walking, swimming, or yoga are all enjoyable activities that may help you burn calories and improve your overall health. Aim for at least 30 minutes of moderate-intensity exercise most days of the week to help with weight reduction or maintenance.

Preventing Cancer Recurrence With Diet

While food alone cannot prevent cancer recurrence, following a healthy eating pattern may help with overall cancer care. Consume a range of nutrient-dense meals to offer your body the vitamins, minerals, and antioxidants it needs to maintain immunological function and attack cancer cells.

Including enough fruits and vegetables in your diet is essential. These foods have high levels of antioxidants, which help protect cells from free radical damage and may lower the chance of cancer recurrence. Aim for a rainbow of colors on your plate, since each fruit and vegetable has distinct health advantages.

Whole grains, lean meats, and healthy fats should all be cornerstones in your diet. Whole grains include fiber, which assists digestion and regulates blood sugar levels. Lean proteins including chicken, fish, beans, and lentils provide critical amino acids for cell repair and immunological function. Nuts, seeds, avocados, and olive oil provide healthy fats, which may help decrease inflammation and promote heart health.

Establishing A Lifelong Healthy Eating Pattern

Individuals with lung cancer must adopt a healthy eating pattern for the rest of their lives to maintain their general health and well-being. Instead of considering dietary changes as transient, aim to develop long-term lifestyle changes that prioritize healthy meals and mindful eating practices.

The Mediterranean diet is one method for establishing a healthy eating pattern, emphasizing plant-based foods, whole grains, lean meats, and healthy fats. This method has been linked to several health advantages, including a lower risk of cancer, heart disease, and other chronic illnesses.

In addition to concentrating on particular meals, consider your eating patterns and behaviors. Savor each mouthful, chew gently, and be aware of hunger and fullness signs. Avoid distractions when eating, such as television or technological gadgets, to encourage conscious intake and reduce overeating.

Regular Follow-Ups With A Dietitian

Individuals with lung cancer need regular follow-ups with a dietician to obtain personalized dietary recommendations and support throughout their treatment and recovery journey. A dietitian can assist you with navigating dietary changes, addressing nutritional problems, and optimizing your eating plan to fit your specific health requirements.

During follow-up sessions, your dietitian will evaluate your food consumption, monitor your weight and nutritional status, and provide personalized suggestions to help you improve your overall health and wellness. They may also assist you with any treatment-related side effects, such as lack of appetite, taste changes, or digestive concerns, by prescribing nutrient-dense meals and meal planning tactics.

Diet Changes To Meet Changing Health Needs

As your cancer treatment progresses, it is critical that you alter your diet to meet your changing nutritional requirements. Whether you're in treatment, remission, or transitioning to survivorship, working closely with a dietician may assist ensure that your nutritional plan is optimized to support your health and well-being at every stage.

If you encounter changes in appetite, taste, or digestion after treatment, your dietician may assist you in identifying nutrient-dense meals that are both soft on your stomach and attractive to your palette. They may also give you practical advice on how to deal with side effects and eat properly to help you recover.

As you transition to survivorship, your dietitian can assist you in achieving long-term health objectives like as maintaining a healthy weight, lowering the risk of cancer recurrence, and improving overall well-being via dietary and lifestyle changes. Regular follow-ups with your dietician will ensure that your food plan is still suited to your specific requirements and preferences as you go beyond cancer treatment.

CONCLUSION

To summarise, although food alone cannot prevent or cure lung cancer, eating a good diet may improve general health and may help with disease management. A diet high in fruits, vegetables, whole grains, lean meats, and healthy fats may supply critical nutrients and antioxidants that support the immune system while also reducing inflammation and oxidative stress.

Furthermore, avoiding or restricting processed foods, sugary drinks, red and processed meats, and excessive alcohol use might reduce possible risk factors for lung cancer and improve health outcomes.

Individuals diagnosed with lung cancer must collaborate closely with their healthcare team, including trained dietitians, to design a personalized nutrition plan based on their unique requirements and treatment regimen.

This may include treating treatment-related adverse effects such as lack of appetite, weight loss, or trouble swallowing, as well as developing ways to maintain enough nutrition throughout the cancer journey.

Overall, although dietary choices are just one part of lung cancer care, they may supplement medical therapy and improve the quality of life for those impacted by the illness. More study on the effect of food on lung cancer prevention and treatment is needed to better understand its potential influence and improve supportive care measures.

THE END